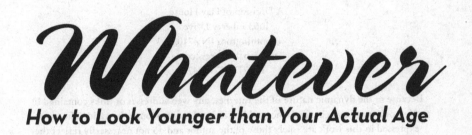

Whatever

How to Look Younger than Your Actual Age

TRICIA BUENVENIDA

BALBOA.PRESS
A DIVISION OF HAY HOUSE

Balboa Press books may be ordered through booksellers or by contacting:

Balboa Press
A Division of Hay House
1663 Liberty Drive
Bloomington, IN 47403
www.balboapress.com
1 (877) 407-4847

Because of the dynamic nature of the Internet, any web addresses or links contained in
this book may have changed since publication and may no longer be valid. The views
expressed in this work are solely those of the author and do not necessarily reflect the
views of the publisher, and the publisher hereby disclaims any responsibility for them.

The author of this book does not dispense medical advice or prescribe the use of any
technique as a form of treatment for physical, emotional, or medical problems without the
advice of a physician, either directly or indirectly. The intent of the author is only to offer
information of a general nature to help you in your quest for emotional and spiritual well-
being. In the event you use any of the information in this book for yourself, which is your
constitutional right, the author and the publisher assume no responsibility for your actions.

Any people depicted in stock imagery provided by Getty Images are models,
and such images are being used for illustrative purposes only.
Certain stock imagery © Getty Images.

Interior Image Credit: Yvette Martins

THE HOLY BIBLE, NEW INTERNATIONAL VERSION®, NIV® Copyright © 1973,
1978, 1984, 2011 by Biblica, Inc.® Used by permission. All rights reserved worldwide.

English Standard Version (ESV)
The Holy Bible, English Standard Version. ESV® Text Edition: 2016. Copyright
© 2001 by Crossway Bibles, a publishing ministry of Good News Publishers.

Print information available on the last page.

ISBN: 978-1-9822-4517-7 (sc)
ISBN: 978-1-9822-4518-4 (e)

Balboa Press rev. date: 05/05/2020

Dedication

For Jax. May you always have a youthful, kind, and loving heart.

CONTENTS

Acknowledgements ix

Foreword xi

Chapter 1   Meditate 1

Chapter 2   Take Care of Your Skin 5

Chapter 3   Eliminate Envy 10

Chapter 4   Act How You Feel 14

Chapter 5   Laugh and Be Joyful 18

Chapter 6   Exercise Regularly 22

Chapter 7   Eat Well 25

Chapter 8   Get Your Sleep 29

Chapter 9   Choose Good Friends 31

Chapter 10 Pick the Right Partner 35

Chapter 11 Embrace Motherhood 38

Chapter 12 Take the Risk 42

Chapter 13 Tackle Your Fears 47

Chapter 14 Love Who You Are 51

Chapter 15 Enjoy Your Work 54

Chapter 16 Believe 58

Chapter 17 Give, Give, and Give Some More 61

Chapter 18 Whatever 65

Conclusion 69

Appendix 71

ACKNOWLEDGEMENTS

There are quite a few people I want to thank for the publication of this book. Of course, I owe so much to my family: Ry, Jax, my mom, my sister Pearl, my brother RJ, and all of my wonderful aunts, uncles, and cousins. It is because of them that I am confident to try new things. I also want to acknowledge my in-laws for their never-ending love and support: Bruce, Joanne, Sam, and Taj.

Thank you also to my dear, loving friends who have either supported me, inspired me, or read countless versions of this book (in no particular order): Chris and Angie De Oliveira, Janine Sagar, Maria Wallin, Erik Svensson, Yvette Martins, Cindy Tidler, Hang Leibold, Aren Anderson, Renee Lerneby, John and Veronica Cavebring, Chris Barry, Sylvia Read, Lisa Sanders, Shannon Holbert, Julia Crighton, Angela Busby, Anna Quanne, Vlad Coho, Paul Farina, Craig Hazenfield, Leigh Ann Pena, Jennifer Nguyen, Aubrey Reavis, Hanh Tran, Eve Donovan, Anne Foreman, Jeff Anglada, Cara Haleblian, Amanda Brown, Peter Panagopoulos, Zachary Prell, Meesh Pierce, and Maripat Bacalzo.

Finally, thank you to my Dad. I miss you every day.

FOREWORD

Almost 10 years ago, I started writing a blog, www.nouglyduckling. com. I initially started it because I wanted my college roommate Janine, who is one of my very best friends and is always in the know of what is cool and cutting edge, to help me write it and share her secrets and insights. Unfortunately, she became too busy with both personal and work commitments. Since I had already established the platform, I decided to continue without her and thus my blog began.

Through the years, doing that blog has confirmed my love of writing which I've always known since childhood. For me, nothing sorts out my thoughts more clearly.

So, I write and write and write all the time. Not one day goes by that I do not write. Of course, I write for my marketing clients, but I also write for my family, my friends, and myself.

So now, here is my biggest writing undertaking to date. It came about because my dear friend Angie suggested that I should start telling people how I maintain my youthful looks and attitude. This suggestion comes after countless people have also asked me about the same.

Initially, I was hesitant to do this because I really never think about my age: 49. Putting it to paper gives it some serious credence, and I never want to be confined by those parameters. Even seeing it written in black and white is unsettling.

Also, for me, it seems so egocentric to be writing "my beauty secrets." There are lots of incredibly beautiful people that are my age or even older: Halle Berry, Jennifer Aniston, Angela Bassett, Christie Brinkley, and Jennifer Lopez, just to name a few.

But I am earnestly removing my ego in the hopes that some of these "secrets" may actually help someone.

Obviously a lot of it is genetic. I don't know why I don't have one strand of gray hair, but my mom at 76 doesn't have any gray hair either. I'm also, thankfully, not yet in need of bi-focals or readers.

I'm also Filipino. As the saying goes, "Asian don't raisin." According to an AARP article I read, "youthful bodies may be thin, but youthful faces have fat. The rosy cheeks of a baby are full" and Asians have a wider bone structure than a typical Caucasian face. So, thanks to my fat face I don't have to inject fillers.

I kid, but I can also credit a lot of my "plastic-surgery/filler/botox-free," younger-looking life to some specific habits.

So, here is how I live my life. I am not saying this is the best way to live your life, or even how you should live your life. This is merely an account of how I live my life. I am still learning, too, but this is what I have found works best for me.

I hope parts of it will inspire and help you. I believe our biggest purpose is to serve others so that's what I am aiming to do.

Thank you for reading.

1

Meditate

"Praying is talking to the Universe. Meditation is listening to it." - Paulo Coelho

IN 2015, I STARTED TO BE very serious about meditating. The mind is very powerful and if you can tame the chatter in your head, I believe you can achieve all things.

So every morning, without fail, I meditate for 10 minutes. Some days I can carve out time to do it for longer, but most days, it is 10 minutes and then I begin my day.

I can honestly say that I have seen a drastic change on how I live my life because of my regular meditation habit. It wasn't a sudden transformation but remember, I have now been faithfully meditating for almost 5 years. Slowly but surely, I am more conscious and self-aware of how my mind works, and I try to function at my highest level at all times.

To me, operating at the highest level means creating a positive, grand life. By doing so, I make a concerted effort to tune out any negative or fear-based thoughts and instead, come from a place of love and generosity. It also means that I take full responsibility for my life.

I know that where I am in my life is because I have made choices that have led me here.

Studies state that meditation may help develop a stronger understanding of self, help you grow into your best self, and develop a greater understanding of how you relate to those around you. From my experience, I believe this is true.

I also recently read a *Forbes* article on how meditation helps preserve the aging brain. A UCLA study found that long-term meditators had better-preserved brains than non-meditators as they aged. Findings showed that participants who'd been meditating for an average of 20 years had more gray matter volume throughout the brain.[1]

If that is true, then that is another factor that keeps me youthful.

If you are new to meditating, or have never tried it, don't be scared. I suggest you put yourself in a quiet room, and make sure you are comfortable with your back propped up. I like to meditate on my bed with pillows behind me. I use the Calm app and set it to the timed 10-minute or 15-minute meditation but Calm makes it easy to use any of their guided meditations.

Once you are comfortable, just slowly breathe in and out and try to follow your breath and avoid any distractions. This is easier said than done, but the goal is to try to get your mind in a neutral state so that it is relaxed.

Honestly, most of the time, my meditation sessions just set me up to have a calm, relaxed mind for the day, but on a couple occasions, I have been able to be fully in the zone and achieve a trance-like state and actually manifest tangible desires.

Regardless, doing any meditation should help you find more peace and clarity, and maybe inspire some creativity. Start with five minutes

---

[1] Walton, Alice. "7 Ways Meditation Can Actually Change the Brain." *Forbes*, 9 Feb 2015.

and then build from there, and then be consistent. Choose the same time of day so it is part of your regular routine.

Sometimes at night, I will also listen to Wayne Dyer's meditation, "Three Magic Words," just before I go to sleep. I am still learning about energy vibration but this particular meditation is very calming and helps reinforce the living of a stress-free, tranquil life so that we can vibrate at our highest level. My goal is to consistently operate at this high level because it is when we are living in this high energy that we can be fully alive and on purpose.

The one big thing I absolutely believe, believe, believe in is that how you are feeling on the inside – the mental, spiritual, and emotional side of yourself – will manifest on the outside, or physical part of you.

Your outer world is merely a reflection of your inner world.

I believe that if you consciously monitor your thoughts, you have the ability to:

1) Control your thoughts
2) Remove your thoughts
3) Install any thought

My greatest power is my ability to choose my own thoughts.

At the end of the book, I've shared a bunch of books and incredibly inspiring quotes that I like to reference on how to think. The mind is a powerful organ so we must learn to use it to help us, not limit us.

Feel free to bookmark these quotes as mantras, or even memorize one. I think mastering the mind is one of the most important accomplishments anyone can achieve in their lifetime.

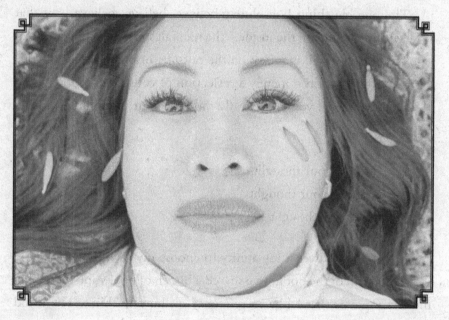

2

Take Care of Your Skin

"The best foundation you can wear is glowing, healthy
skin." - Anonymous

I STARTED MY CAREER IN THE BEAUTY industry. When I graduated
from Boston University, I followed my close friends from Boston
to New York City with the hopes of securing an advertising account
management job.

I found it at Grey Advertising on the Procter & Gamble Eurocos
account, which was their European fragrances division. I remember
often sitting in the production and editing rooms for hours adding
all these different store tags (e.g., "Available at Dillard's") to the same
Laura Biagiotti or Hugo Boss spot. Ahh, such fond memories.

From there, I was promoted to Cover Girl's advertising account
and to this day, that group of colleagues are the most creative people
I have ever met in my life. The head of the creative team was Dick
Huebner, who discovered Christie Brinkley!

I would be involved in print and television shoots with a Cover
Girl model like Niki Taylor and recognized that, yes, she was
physically beautiful, but it was her inner confidence that made her
a Cover Girl.

When I moved to Tarlow Advertising, the agency that had the Victoria's Secret advertising account, I was privileged to work with such a small team. Due to its size, I was given the responsibility to manage and have an impact on Victoria's Secret's advertising strategy, even as a 25-year old. I want to thank Dick Tarlow and Nancy Brodsky for this experience because it was them, and Carol Clark, our Creative Director, (and of course VS President Ed Razek) who created the now iconic Angels campaign. Oh gosh how I wish I had those original storyboards!

I remember going from photo shoot to photo shoot, and oftentimes I would have to pick up supermodel Stephanie Seymour from her home in Connecticut prior to the shoot.

Of course, Stephanie Seymour is absolutely gorgeous but I witnessed firsthand how she transformed from being merely a lowkey, pretty lady sitting in the back seat with me, to stepping out of the car and literally becoming a fabulous Victoria's Secret supermodel. Again, it was that something special inside her.

In fact, all of those original Victoria's Secret Angels supermodels –Tyra Banks, Helena Christensen, Karen Mulder, Daniela Pestova, and Stephanie Seymour - had that "it" factor so beautifully captured by the incredibly talented Herb Ritts.

I recount my early career days because those were some of the most glamorous days of my life. I was in my early 20s, living in Manhattan, and going to photo shoots with beautiful supermodels, working with talented makeup artists such as Pat McGrath and Brigitte Reiss Andersen, and shooting with phenomenal photographers and directors like Herb Ritts, Gilles Bensimon, and Walter Chin.

It was also then that I realized the importance of beauty, cosmetics, and proper skincare.

To have good skin, one must absolutely wash one's face and take care of it.

So, what do I do? It is so crazy simple but here it is:

Morning Routine:

1) First, I use a gentle cleanser to wash my face. I usually use a pea-sized drop of Cetaphil or Glossier's Milky Jelly Cleanser, but if I am gifted a cleanser, I will often use those, too.
2) Then I put on facial sunscreen with a minimum SPF 15. Again, I am not particular about the brand, although I gravitate towards French brands like L'Oreal, Caudalie, or La Roche-Posay. However, recently, I've been using Arbonne's RE9 Advanced Protecting Cream with SPF 15.
3) I put Vaseline on my lips so they aren't dry.

Voila! I'm done. I will then apply makeup (or not) and am ready to go out for the day.

Evening Routine:

1) Again, I use a drop of cleanser to clear my face of any makeup debris.
2) Then I will put on an eye cream. I am not loyal to any brand but the ones I've been using lately are Restorsea's Revitalizing Eye Cream (my friend Patti Pao's company), Caudalie Vine(Activ), or a brandless eye cream with argan oil that I recently bought when I was in Marrakech, Morocco.
3) Then, I put on an evening moisturizer. Currently I'm using Amala's Advanced Firming Complex (I was helping this brand with their marketing and gifted this item) and I really like it. However, if I feel like my skin is particularly dry and needs some hydration, I will use a facial oil such as a rosehip oil. I also

like Nivea's Hyaluron Cellular Filler, which is reputed to be a cheaper version of Crème de la Mer.

4) Finally, I put Vaseline on my lips so they aren't dry.

I often switch it up with my brands and formulas since I, always the marketer and consumer, like to discover new products. But, above is essentially my daily routine.

About twice a week, I will use my Clarisonic facial brush in the shower to exfoliate and remove dead skin cells.

Also, every month or so, I make sure to do a scrub and mask of some sort (lately I've been using Avene's Gentle Exfoliating Scrub and Caudalie's Glycolic Peel Mask).

With regards to body, I always moisturize after I shower. These days, I use pure coconut oil but I will use any body lotion as long as my skin is not dry. If I find my skin is dry during the day, I will make sure to reapply coconut oil or lotion. I am especially vigilant about hand lotion. The best I found is L'Occitane's Shea Butter Hand Cream. Anytime I wash my hands, I will apply some lotion afterwards because our hands are the first telltale sign of age.

Finally, I am very diligent about getting a facial every month. I think it is very important to have your face massaged as it improves skin circulation. Here in Portugal, I faithfully go to Claudia Ferreira of Cátia e Cláudia Salon who will infuse Vitamin C if needed or maybe some glycolic acid. In California, I have my facialists Simi Gholamabbas and Judy Small to thank for their diligence and expertise.

As you can see, I have been religious about applying sunscreen on my face for YEARS – since my 20s. Most Asians don't want to have dark skin, and in the Philippine culture, mestizo and mestiza looks with the ideal café au lait complexion are very revered. Also, in my case, I learned early on, just from working in the beauty business, that sunscreen prevents wrinkles and age spots.

Plus, I always wash my face and apply generous amounts of moisturizer or even oil before I go to bed. I don't ever wear foundation or any coverage cream that could block my pores. Finally, I am not a smoker and I never ever wear makeup when I work out, knowing that I will likely sweat. Not even lipstick.

But most importantly, I try not to hold anything inside. I seriously believe that toxicity becomes cancer or morphs into some other disease, and it will certainly age you and show up on your skin.

3

Eliminate Envy

"The wicked envy and hate; it is their way of admiring." –
Victor Hugo

FOR THOSE OF YOU WHO FAITHFULLY read my blog, I wrote that my biggest secret to staying youthful is to be happy and kind. This is true, but I wanted to actually expand on it by saying that jealousy, envy, and competition does not have a home in a loving and peaceful heart.

When you are not centered, calm, and at peace, I believe you open yourself up to premature aging.

I don't know about you but I see this aging in the faces of people I know who are envious and competitive. They may try to conceal it, but their skin does not glow! It is because the light inside of them is not bright. I honestly and sincerely believe this and see it firsthand.

Really! Our bodies are merely vessels for the light inside all of us. I always know when I am with someone who does not truly want the best for me. I feel it in their energy. I'm sure many of you have encountered the same.

I find that these very competitive people are constantly trying to outbest everyone, and the whole world, including people they call their friends, is their competition. They believe they need to be better than anyone in everything they do to feel superior and good about themselves, and I find this energy to be very narcissistic and selfish.

So, it is especially prudent for us to guard our heart and light and limit contact with people who do not want the best for it. As I say, it is best to love them from afar.

I particularly like this Bible passage from Proverbs 4:23-26 (NIV):

23 Above all else, guard your heart,

for everything you do flows from it.

24 Keep your mouth free of perversity;

keep corrupt talk far from your lips.

25 Let your eyes look straight ahead;

fix your gaze directly before you.

26 Give careful thought to the paths for your feet

and be steadfast in all your ways.

Life is very short and there is nothing stopping you from living the life you want to live. Rest in the assurance that you can do it and don't worry about the haters.

What does your dream life look like? If you can envision it, then you can go after it.

Tune out the noise, try to stay centered and calm, and enjoy this adventure called life, with all its ups and downs included.

Stay focused on that vision and don't mind what others will think. Believe me, not everyone is on my side. I wish that were the case but it isn't. Sadly, I have learned that there will always be people who will speak negatively about me and there is not much I can do about it.

On the flip side, don't worry about how others are living their lives. Recognize that these others are (hopefully) also on their specific path to fulfillment and just love and accept them for who they are. Sometimes this is best done at a distance.

One of my life's hardest lessons was to learn that not everyone will want the best for me. I remember crying in college to my friend Janine when I realized that there were people who did not want me to succeed. I naively thought that we all cheered for everyone. My once-innocent self shockingly learned that there are people who will deliberately sabotage someone's pathway to success if they feel it will impede theirs.

There are also some people who like to gossip and always find some reason to speak negatively about people.

But I realize that this negative attitude is more a reflection of that person and his or her insecurities. It always surprises me when I believe someone has his or her act together and then I hear them speak poorly of another person. Hmmm. Why do you care so much about that other person? Could it be that they somehow bring about inadequacies about yourself?

When I find that I am envying someone, it is usually due to an insecurity on my part. It is then that I take a step back and remember that I can achieve whatever that person has attained, too. If that person achieved it, what is stopping me from doing the same? Nothing! Just my limiting belief. So, I celebrate that person even more, and move forward with the confidence that if that person did it, so can I. I put out positive energy so it will come back to me.

Here's my foolproof method to CALM down when I find myself harboring any jealous feelings:

Catch yourself when you are feeling jealous

Acknowledge and be aware of what may be triggering this envy

Let go of any limiting beliefs

Move forward knowing you are strong and secure in yourself and your abilities

We all have our own specific talents gifted to us by the Universe. As the saying goes: "A flower does not think of competing to the flower next to it, it just blooms." That is our ultimate purpose – to become the most beautiful flower we can be. Think how absolutely gorgeous this world will be when all these beautiful flowers in the field meet their full potential, too.

4

Act How You Feel

"The secret of staying young is to live honestly, eat slowly, and lie about your age." – Lucille Ball

I JEST BUT I DON'T. THAT LUCILLE Ball quote is great. Unfortunately, society has placed a stigma on aging, and I understand. As we get older, for the most part, we don't have the same attitude on life. It is a function of experience. I am not as naïve as I once was so often it looks like cynicism.

Also, my body is not the same. It has had many more years of steering the ship, and like a car, the wear and tear on my body makes it less efficient. When I veer off my regular exercise regimen (like the week between Christmas and New Year's Day), sadly I do feel stiffness in the morning that I never had in my 20s.

We envy youth because they represent vigor and a joie de vivre. Youth are more likely to have a carefree attitude and have fun, they are adventurous and like to explore and experience new things. But most of all, youth have hope because they are excited about their futures.

Once we get to middle age, a lot of this youthful outlook may be lost because of the idea that there is not much left of this future. Or, we just have too many responsibilities that make us less carefree.

So, I don't think about my actual age. Really. I never even think about it. Age is really just a number. In fact, I often forget how old I am because I don't give it much priority.

It reminds me of the guru character in the book *Eat, Pray, Love*, who doesn't know his actual age and states a different number according to how he is feeling that day.

Science has proved that everyone ages at a different rate. Some people seem to age very rapidly —in terms of health and appearance— while others age more slowly.

In recent years, studies have shown that our biological age is often a more reliable indicator of future health than our actual age.[2] I've read that using our biological age as a benchmark may even allow us to slow – or reverse – the aging process.

Reverse? OK. Maybe it is possible. So, I've stopped focusing on my actual age and am just living my life. If you were 15, 21, or 25 years old, what would you want to do? Do it. Don't let age hold you back. Act as if you are that age and live life at that age.

I'm often told I have a childlike quality, but it is because I don't feel any different than I did when I was much younger. I just experience life with the same wonder and curiosity, and maybe some naivety, because there is always something new and original to discover every day. Why would I act any differently now?

Seriously, do you feel any different from December 31 of the year before and January 1 of the new year? Unless you really partied it up, probably no. This is the same type of scenario.

Sometimes I feel that I am still in high school. I went to an all-girls' private Catholic high school and although it was a wonderful education, because of that, I missed out on many typical high school

---

[2] Thomson, Helen. "Why Your Real Age May Be Older – Or Younger – Than Your Years." *New Scientist,* 28 June 2017.

experiences and so I love watching movies targeted to that age group or even reading Young Adult novels.

It is likely because I missed out on being in a classroom with boys and experiencing some of those stereotypical teen things – during those pivotal teen years – that I wish I could relive them now.

Silly, I know, but in my head, I am 16.

Other times, I am 28, just recently graduated from grad school and going full force at my career as a newly initiated MBA graduate with lots of ideas and energy.

Since that's how old I feel, that's how old I am, and I don't give it much thought.

If you are one of those people who is hung up on age (it *is* hard to dismiss with societal pressures), try and remember that your biological age is more indicative than actual age. Try not to look at your actual age as anything more than any other number that identifies you such as a social security number or passport number so you don't place any emotion on it. And then live life at the age you believe you are.

I live my life how I feel inside, and that is one way I stay young.

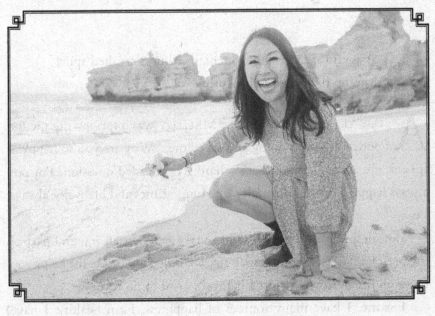

17

5

Laugh and Be Joyful

"A joyful heart is good medicine, but a crushed spirit dries up the bones." (Proverbs 17:22, ESV)

A FEW YEARS AGO, MY FRIEND MALLORY was interviewing me for a podcast she was doing and asked me, "Why are you so happy?" It took me aback because that's a hard, very loaded question. I'm not always happy - I do go through some tough times and life is not always easy.

But, despite this, I always try to make laughter an integral part of my personality. Many sources say that making a gratitude list helps you focus on the positive. I guess I naturally tend to do this.

For me, I have many sources of happiness. I am healthy. I have a supportive, stable, and loving family. I enjoy what I do as a job and love working and helping my clients succeed. I have wonderful, positive friends. I am currently living abroad in Portugal and prior to COVID-19, was traveling a lot. I am not struggling financially.

I do want to address that last point because I want to be sympathetic to those who struggle with money. Money does buy happiness and comfort, but it is only to a certain point. In my case, I've never had to worry about where my next meal is coming from, I've had all the resources of the First World available to me, and I've never had to do the type of manual labor that lowers life expectancy. This book is not targeted to those facing those kinds of circumstances. I feel fortunate that I hit the life lottery.

I am not saying that my life is all roses, but I hate seeing quotes or memes that say something similar to "Everyone you meet is fighting a battle you know nothing about. Be kind. Always."

I disagree. I agree with being kind always, but not everyone is fighting a battle. I am not fighting a battle.

I mean, I try every day to become a better version of myself, and as I said in Chapter 1, I try and control my thoughts so I choose not to be in turmoil about something in my life.

On the contrary, I always try to be really JOYFUL.

As you may have already deduced, I am a big believer. God, Universe, Energy, Karma. Whatever you want to call it, I believe in it.

I grew up in a Catholic household and my family is very devout. Although I may not subscribe to all the tenets, Catholicism has proven to be a very solid base for me, and I feel very much at home when I step into a Catholic mass, wherever it is in the world. So, I am faithful about attending mass every Sunday, even here in Portugal where I don't understand the majority of what they are saying since I don't speak Portuguese.

From a very early age, I felt God/Universe/Spirit's presence in my life and I believe that the Universe wants us to be happy. The Universe has gifted us with so much and we are all so lucky to be experiencing it.

So, I work very hard to be joyful and try to laugh about something every day. Even when things don't go my way or I'm frustrated or sad about a situation, I try to find the lesson and the silver lining. I want to be positive and happy because that energy rubs off on other people, and makes them positive and happy.

In fact, I think comedians are amazing. My favorites like Ellen

DeGeneres, Tiffany Haddish, Ali Wong, and Hassan Minhaj are blessed with the talent to make others laugh and feel great. Wow - what an amazing gift!

Since I can't do this, I aim to be happy. I try not to complain because I want others to be happy around me. Really, all I want is for everyone to be happy. I believe that if you come from a place of happiness and love, you can accomplish more and be in a position of strength to help others.

To quote New York Times bestselling author and motivational speaker Gabby Bernstein, "The more joyful we are, the more light we shine on the world, the more power we have to express our presence, and the more positive energy we put out."

As I said in Chapter 1, we vibrate at our highest level when we are living joyfully, and I want to consistently operate at this high level because this is when we are most creative, innovative, and in tune with the Universe.

For those of you who need help finding laughter, I recommend that you watch or listen to some stand-up. I remember when I was pregnant with my son Jax, I would watch a lot of stand-up comedy. Or, I would listen to a comedy playlist on Spotify when I did a walk around the neighborhood.

I had read that laughter is so important for your baby in utero so I wanted to make sure I would laugh – hard core belly laugh - a lot and every day while I was pregnant. There are so many talented comedians so there is a plethora of specials to watch, and I find that just listening or watching them perform can change my ho-hum mood to one of happiness and positivity.

If you are in a funky mood, download "Comedy Top Tracks" from Spotify and listen to a few of the spots. I guarantee it will put you in a better disposition. I find that not only is the comedian funny but the audience laughter is contagious.

Finally, I believe that if you help others achieve their own joy, it will increase yours. Joy is here to be shared. I believe that the more sincerely joyful you are for others and their accomplishments, the more the Universe rewards you.

I know full-time happiness is unrealistic and can't happen all the time but I live my life so that for me, joy is the majority of my time.

6

Exercise Regularly

"Take care of your body. It's the only place you have to live." – Jim Rohn

I WON'T GO INTO MUCH DETAIL ABOUT this because I'm sure all of you already know that regular exercise does a body good.

Numerous studies have shown that physical exercise has been well demonstrated as an effective anti-aging intervention.[3] In this particular study I cite, it states that physical exercise has an anti-aging effect on the hippocampus region of the brain, which controls memory, learning, and balance.

I was also recently binge-watching Netflix's The Goop Lab series and in the "Health-Span Plan" episode which explores the science of antiaging, Gwyneth Paltrow and members of her team speak with Valter Longo, who is the director of the University of Southern California's Longevity Institute. Longo noted that we should be doing 150 minutes of exercise per week for maximum longevity.

---

[3] Garatachea, N., Santos-Lozano, A., Hughes, D.C., Gomez-Cabello, A., 2017, Physical Exercise as an Effective Antiaging Intervention, 2017 March 29 <https://doi.org/10.1155/2017/7317609>.

If you are one of those people who can't seem to ever fit exercise into your daily routine, I suggest you schedule it like any other appointment or meeting you may have on your calendar.

That is seriously how I stay disciplined enough to work out 4–5 days per week, if not more. It has merely become part of my routine, like brushing my teeth twice a day.

Also, I don't believe exercise has to be really strenuous. Even Longo noted that the important thing is not the actual exercise you are doing, but the routine physical activity. My professional fitness instructor friends will probably disagree with me, but I think that if you can manage to find 30 minutes a day to do a brisk walk, you are consistently exercising.

My activities of choice are yoga, padel (a sport very popular here in Portugal), running, and weights. I definitely don't have my 20-year old body, but I am healthy, strong, and active so my body functions as it should.

In case you are interested, here is my weekly routine:

Monday: 1 hour padel, 80 minutes Vinyasa yoga
Tuesday: 40 minutes horseback riding
Wednesday: 80 minutes Vinyasa yoga
Thursday: 45 minutes running, weights, and stretching
Friday: 80 minutes Vinyasa yoga
Saturday: 30 minutes running and/or weights and stretching

Of course, it varies from time to time and I'm not always so disciplined, but this is what it is for the most part.

If you are not yet an avid exerciser, start with 20-minute walks every other day. I like to listen to a podcast or some upbeat music so I lose track of time and before I know it, the 20-minute walk is done. With exercise, consistency is key.

Most importantly, I don't need to take prescription medications to control my blood pressure, sugar levels, cholesterol levels, or heart rate. In fact, I hardly ever take any medications at all. Isn't this what we all want?

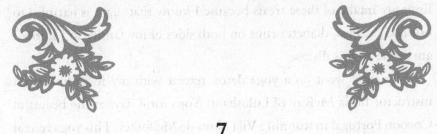
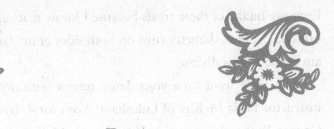

7

Eat Well

"Don't dig your grave with your own knife and fork." -
Old English Proverb

IN CONJUNCTION WITH EXERCISE, I TRY to be very mindful of what I put in my body.

What you eat hugely affects your health. If you eat healthy foods, you'll feel better, stronger, have more energy, and likely live longer.

My cousin-in-law Rachel wrote a very great, insightful piece, "24 Things I have Learned at 24" and one of her 24 points is: "Eating healthy and taking care of yourself is a form of self-respect. You do not have to apologize for it."

She said it so eloquently that I am just repeating it.

This bible passage from 1 Corinthians 6:19-20 (NIV) also provides a similar teaching: "Do you not know that your bodies are temples of the Holy Spirit, who is in you, whom you have received from God? You are not your own; you were bought at a price. Therefore honor God with your bodies."

So, I try not to abuse my body by smoking or choosing poor food choices. It is incredibly difficult. I love sugar and cookies, pastries, pies, and cakes are definitely my indulgence. Regardless, I try very hard to limit my intake of these treats because I know that sugar is harmful to our bodies. Plus, diabetes runs on both sides of my family so I know I am prone to this disease.

I recently went on a yoga detox retreat with my incredible yoga instructor Luisa McKay of Lulushanti Yoga for 4 days at the beautiful Cocoon Portugal in stunning Vila Nova de Melfontes. This yoga retreat was very eye-opening for me because we really did a hard-core food detox. We only had vegetable juices for breakfast and lunch, and a vegetable soup for dinner. No caffeine, salt, or sugar.

Luckily for me, I don't regularly drink coffee anymore so I did not have any coffee withdrawal symptoms (although I had a horrible headache for a week straight when I first cut it cold turkey three years ago).

But the more astounding result of this detox was that I actually had more energy and focus when on this limited vegetable diet.

After speaking with Sharon Sinclair, our retreat nutritionist and now my nutritionist, I knew I had to change my diet and increase my vegetable intake. Now, I try to make vegetables the majority of what is on my plate.

What else? I've been dairy-free for a while now due to a lactose intolerance and recently, per Sharon's suggestion, I also eliminated gluten from my diet.

I am not a professional nutritionist so I can't speak expertly on why removing gluten from your diet can help avoid the triggering of autoimmune diseases and inflammation of the gut. What I can tell you is that I have absolutely noticed a difference since I've removed gluten from my diet – I'm hardly ever bloated, my stomach rarely bothers me, and I have a lot more energy.

Sharon sent me a great paleo seed bread recipe from award winning Nutritional Therapist, Functional Nutrition Practitioner and UK Chef

Christine Bailey[4]. One loaf of bread includes ground-up almonds, flax seeds, chia seeds, sesame seeds, and arrowroot powder, and it only takes about 30 minutes to make.

It is so delicious and I use it for my sandwiches or eat it as a morning snack with almond butter. By the way, I also saw that 74-year old fashion designer Norma Kamali (who looks incredible!) recently posted her seed bread recipe on her Instagram page, too. Frankly, she is incredibly inspirational and swears by seed bread, so give it a try.

I also try to intermittent fast every now and then. For those unfamiliar with intermittent fasting, it merely means that I do not eat anything for 16 hours. So, if last night I finished my dinner at 6pm, I won't eat anything until today at 10am. Many do intermittent fasting for weight loss, but since I have managed to keep a stable weight all my life, I do it for the health benefits: lowering insulin levels and increasing fat-burning hormones, and thus creating better metabolism.

I've never been much of an alcoholic drinker, but I may have something at a party, so probably about 15-20 glasses per year.

I do, however, drink plenty of water. Water is my beverage of choice – nothing quenches my thirst more than water. Health authorities commonly recommend eight 8-ounce glasses, which equals about 2 liters, or half a gallon.[5] I pretty much consume this amount regularly since most days, all I drink is water.

Also, I pretty much cut out red meat from my diet years ago on advice from an acupuncturist specializing in fertility, and I'm allergic to shellfish so I never eat it. Shellfish may accumulate heavy metals such as mercury or cadmium from their environments, and humans cannot

---

[4] https://www.christinebailey.co.uk/recipe/paleo-seeded-bread/
[5] Gunnars, Kris. "How Much Water Should You Drink Per Day?" *Healthline,* 20 June. 2018.

excrete heavy metals. Over time, this build-up of metals can lead to organ damage and other health issues.[6]

So, what do I do to make healthy eating easier? When I go food shopping, I try and fill my home with healthy nutritious food. It is harder to eat unhealthy food if it is not readily available. Also, I try not to buy processed food.

I am not the best cook, but I cook very simply so I know all the ingredients that go into each dish. Here is an example of one of my day's meals:

> Breakfast: Scrambled eggs with spinach, mushroom, and tomato (cooked in virgin olive oil)
> Lunch: Tuna salad with cucumber, red onion, olives, tomatoes, and avocado with a red wine vinegar and olive oil dressing
> Dinner: Salmon Teriyaki (but instead of Teriyaki sauce, I use Tamari sauce which is gluten-free, or you can make a gluten-free teriyaki sauce), steamed broccoli and carrots, and rice

My friend Janine just tapped me onto a great food delivery service – Daily Harvest. She loves it and as I said in my Foreword, she always knows what is cool and good. I have yet to try it as I'm currently living abroad but it looks like an easy way to add more fruits and vegetables to anyone's diet.

As we know, health is wealth. For me, being healthy gives me energy, vitality, peace, and makes me more confident and comfortable with my body. One of my favorite sayings is "Nothing looks as good as fit feels" and this is absolutely true for me.

---

[6] Losasso, C., Bille, L., Patuzzi, I., Lorenzetto, M., Binato, G., Dalla Pozza, M., Ferre, N., Ricci, A., 2015, Possible Influence of Natural Events on Heavy Metals Exposure From Shellfish Consumption: A Case Study in the North-East of Italy, 2015 Feb. 4 <https://doi.org/10.3389/fpubh.2015.00021>.

8

Get Your Sleep

"Sleep is the best meditation." – Dalai Lama

IF YOU WANT TO REJUVENATE YOUR body, nothing beats sleep. I was listening to my Calm meditation app, and three-time champion and basketball phenom and super philanthropist LeBron James is one of the featured speakers. He dedicates about five minutes on the importance of his sleep routine in order to be the best he can be.

I was so impressed with LeBron's schedule which always includes eight hours of sleep every night, and a two-hour nap during the day.

Sleep is so important for health as we get older. It is the most powerful thing you can do for your health. Sleep has the power to improve your mood, recharge your mind, heal your body, and balance your emotions. It also makes you more creative and productive because you're so much more awake and alert.

Finally, sleep boosts your immune system so you hardly ever get sick, and it is scientifically proven to keep your heart healthy, reduce stress, and may prevent cancer.

I read somewhere that researchers found people who get less than the recommended six to eight hours sleep each night were 12% more likely to die prematurely.[7]

As for me, I need to be better at prioritizing sleep over everything else in life. Although I get six to eight hours sleep regularly, I used to be a very deep, sound sleeper and definitely had my necessary minimum eight hours per night.

Since I became a mom six years ago, I have found that I'm not the sound sleeper I once was. Is it mom instinct?

Regardless, I know that nothing is more valuable to recovery and happiness than sleep so I try to go to bed by 10pm each night.

For some reason, Western society has deemed it ok to go by on four or five hours of sleep per night because it infers that we are being productive and reaching our goals.

But, I believe we need to change this viewpoint. Sleep takes time and that time is necessary for cell regeneration and rejuvenation.

To help me sleep better, I try not to look at any screens one hour before I go to bed. I also turn off the sound on my phone. Better yet, try and charge your phone outside your bedroom. In our home in Portugal, we have blackout screens that pull down that absolutely block out any light so that helps me sleep longer, too.

If you don't have this, buy a sleep mask that will do it. I own a Tempur-Pedic Sleep Mask and I absolutely love it. It is so comfortable and I always use it when I have to fly a red-eye flight. It provides total darkness and I can actually manage to catch a few hours of sleep on a plane.

If you do not get enough sleep, it will definitely age you.

---

[7] "Lack of Sleep 'Linked to Early Death'." *BBC News,* 4 May 2010.

9

Choose Good Friends

"Walk with the wise and become wise; associate with
fools and get in trouble." (Proverbs 13:20, ESV)

THERE ARE QUITE A FEW PASSAGES in the Bible about choosing the
right friends. Life coach Tony Robbins has also said: "The quality
of your life is the quality of your relationships."

I feel very lucky to have an amazing network of friends. My friends
inspire me, help me become the best version of myself, and bring much
support, joy, love, and happiness to my days.

I hope your friends are doing the same for you. If not, why not?

You may have heard the saying "You are the average of the five
people you spend the most time with."

I recently read that social psychologist Dr. David McClelland of
Harvard University studied people and their 'reference groups' over a
30-year period and discovered that the people we habitually associate
with determines as much as 95% of our success or failure in life.[8]

---

[8] McClelland, David C., The Achieving Society (1961). University of Illinois
at Urbana-Champaign's Academy for Entrepreneurial Leadership Historical
Research Reference in Entrepreneurship. Available at SSRN: https://ssrn.com/
abstract=1496181

The people you surround yourself with really matters!

For me, that includes Ry, a life partner who is 10 years younger than me. I will elaborate more on this in the next chapter, but for me, having a younger partner keeps me youthful.

Of course, if your life partner is not 10 years younger than you, it doesn't mean you're going to age more quickly.

But it's good to take account of all of our relationships. Sometimes we have fake or superficial friends. While these acquaintance-type friends can be fun, I try not to make these kinds of people the bulk of my friendships.

Once again, I will reference the Bible with this quote: "But the Lord said to Samuel, "Do not look on his appearance or on the height of his stature, because I have rejected him. For the Lord sees not as man sees: man looks on the outward appearance, but the Lord looks on the heart." (1 Samuel 16:7, ESV)

Throughout my life, I have always tried to choose friends that have a kind, generous heart. In fact, I actually believe that the Universe especially matched Ry and my hearts together.

Making a kind heart my #1 characteristic priority in friendships sometimes means that my friends aren't what society deems the most popular, prettiest, or most financially successful. Yes, sometimes they embody all those things, but sometimes they don't, and for me, it doesn't matter.

So, what if you have a toxic social environment? The first thing to do is limit the amount of time you spend with these negative influences. Cleaning up your friend house will tidy up your mind.

Do not be afraid to place boundaries as it is in your best interest. As I referenced in the Bible passage in Chapter 3, "Above all else, guard your heart, for everything you do flows from it." Of course, always be kind and gracious – but from a distance - knowing that you have to be loving and supportive to yourself first.

I, myself, have done this many times. There have been people in my life that seemed to have my best interest and I would love to hang out with them often, but as time and years went on, I could tell they really were not the kindest friends. So, I slowly pull away from them.

In fact, my dear friend Jen has told me that I fool many people in thinking they can be my best friend but I only let a few people into my inner circle. That is true. I am very selective with my closest friendships, and so should you.

Because of this, I have solid, good, incredibly amazing friends that are family. Oh gosh, I love them so much! To me, they are the most beautiful, wealthiest, and most captivating beings on the planet. I love them because they truly want the best for me, and vice versa. That is true friendship and it most definitely keeps me young.

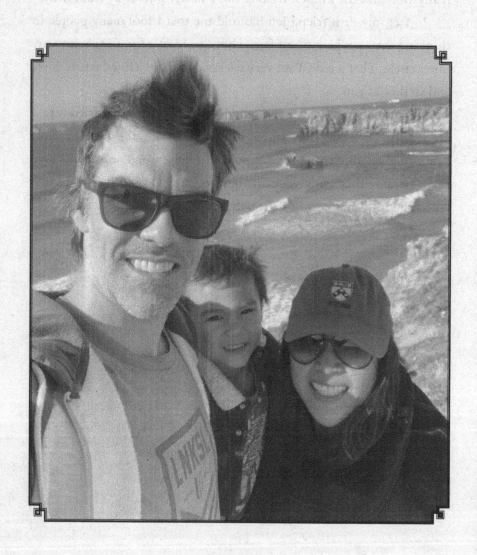

10

Pick the Right Partner

"As iron sharpens iron, so a friend sharpens a friend."
(Proverbs 27:17, ESV)

WHEN I WAS 37, I MET Ry, who was 27. I wasn't planning to be with someone so much younger than me, but we clicked and hit it off immediately. To this day, I tell him that no one communicates with me better than he does.

When I am mad, sad, happy, worried, ecstatic, and everything and all of the above, he will know. I do not hide anything from him.

I hope your significant other acts in the same manner for you, because it is too hard to be anyone except your truest self with your partner.

Before our son Jax was born, Ry and I hardly ever argued. But when we became new parents with little to no sleep, we would have the craziest screaming matches over the littlest things. I don't think I've ever yelled at anyone like that. I can't even imagine if we could not get past these petty arguments.

I can't stress the importance of great communication with your significant other. I believe that if you can communicate properly with each other, you can get through the long haul. One of the main reasons my past relationships did not work out was due to lack of communication.

In my case, Ry is not only my lover and partner, but he is one of my best friends and we can really talk and have great discussions. We are always looking out for each other's best interests.

I saw a meme go around that said: "Fall in love... with someone who is both your safe place and your biggest adventure." When I saw it, I quickly sent it to Ry because that is who he is for me.

Finding the right partner is so important as a stable relationship lends itself to a nurturing environment and sets you both up to become your best and most authentic selves. Stress ages people! Why be with someone who does not honor and support you?

Thankfully, I had a very loving, nurturing father who always wanted the best for me. Because of my Dad, I always knew exactly what I wanted from a love relationship: kindness, respect, authenticity, trust, generosity, and genuine friendship.

I am grateful that I grew up witnessing my parents in a very stable marriage. Although they did argue from time to time, it never entered in my mind they would ever divorce, and they had just celebrated their 45th anniversary when my Dad passed away.

Ry's parents are like this, too. Their relationship, like my parents' relationship, is rock solid, and they recently celebrated 40 years of marriage under their belt.

I absolutely acknowledge that to a certain extent, Ry and I have lived very sheltered, privileged lives to grow up in these kinds of families. But maybe this commonality is why our own relationship is so easy and natural for us.

As they say, I had to kiss a lot of frogs to find my prince. But more importantly, I actually had to learn a lot about myself first — understanding my core values, and what was truly important to me. It is when I found myself that I found Ry.

I wish I could have met him when I was younger, but then he would have been too young for me. So, we met at exactly the right time.

For my friends who are still trying to find that perfect match, don't worry. Do what makes you happy and find joy, and you will see that partner or no partner, you have everything you need.

11

Embrace Motherhood

"There are places in the heart you don't even know exist
until you love a child." – Anne Lamott

I ALMOST DIDN'T INCLUDE THIS CHAPTER BECAUSE it will not apply to
everyone, but it would be an incomplete picture of how I manage
to stay so youthful if I didn't mention it, so here it is.

I've always wanted to be a mom. To me, I don't think there is any
greater blessing than to be able to raise children who will be the next
generation to impact the world.

At 37, when I met Ry, I was a corporate marketing director flying
first class all around the world on behalf of company business.

My job took me to our partners in South Africa and Europe, and
often to Asia at our manufacturing facilities for two-week time spans.
I've lost count of the number of times I've been to Hong Kong and
China and I remember literally living at the Ritz Carlton Hotel in
Seoul, Korea with a regular tailor, hairdresser, masseuse, and nail salon.

I loved my job, I loved traveling, I respected our executive team,
and I loved helping my company succeed. I was indeed living the
glamorous business life.

But, I never forgot about my desire to be a mother.

When I met Ry, I had already been diagnosed with Endometriosis. Apparently, Endometriosis can happen to any menstruating woman but it is more common in women in their 30s and 40s, and you may be more likely to get it if you have never had children.

I remember when my OB/GYN discovered my condition and told me that it was imperative that I pick up a Lupron Depot injection immediately. Lupron Depot suppresses the hormones that cause endometrial tissue to grow and simulates menopause. Unfortunately, there was not one pharmacy in Orange County that carried the injection that day so I had to do a two hour drive up to a specialized pharmacy in Los Angeles. I cried so hard in the car that entire drive up. I was an emotional wreck!

I realized that in my pursuit of fulfilling my professional dreams and goals, I had neglected my personal desires and placed myself in a situation of possible infertility.

But, God was and continues to be so good to me because shortly after this incident is when I met Ry.

When we met, Ry was 27. As I said in the previous chapter, we hit it off right away with an everlasting, strong bond but at that age, he was nowhere ready to be a father. As much as I wanted to have a baby, I knew I couldn't push my timetable on him so I just had to wait and hope. I had to let go of any agendas and remember that the most important thing was that I found someone who I loved and cared about and with whom I enjoyed spending time.

But, luckily for me (and us, really), shortly after he turned 30, Ry told me he was finally ready to be a dad.

So, at 41, I was pregnant!

And my pregnancy was perfect. I didn't have morning sickness at all, and I was pretty upbeat the entire time. I did modify my workouts. Instead of my regular yoga routine, I switched it up to pre-natal yoga, and instead of a regular run, I walked. Obviously, as an older pregnant lady, I was going to be extra careful with myself and my body, but honestly, I can't recall any issues at all. In my memory, it was just an incredible, miraculous time. I think I was just so thrilled to be pregnant that I loved and embraced the entire pregnancy.

So, with this no issue pregnancy, I was ready to deliver via the "Bradley Method." No joke! If you don't know what that is, it is a natural way of childbirth – no drugs needed. Ha! Well, that was clearly wishful thinking on my end.

When my water broke two days before my estimated delivery date, I thought I could breathe right through delivery. Wrong! When my contractions started getting harder, I quickly opted for an epidural. We called my family right away since they would have to fly from Maryland to California, and assumed that by the time they would arrive, little Jax would be in the world.

Wrong again! When my family arrived, I was still going through the contractions. Jax refused to go down my pelvis and my cervix stayed dilated at 9.5 centimeters for the last 6 hours of my 36-hour labor, just short of the 10 centimeters necessary to start pushing.

So, it was an emergency C-section for me. Oh how I cried when the nurse told me that was the plan. But, at that point, I had to surrender, and at the end, I delivered a healthy, happy baby boy.

And this boy truly keeps me youthful. First, babies, toddlers, and kids laugh so much! The littlest thing sets them off with unbridled laughter.

Also, I have a very active boy. I remember doing playdates with other new moms and while their well-behaved daughters were somehow staying still, I had to chase Jax crawling through sofas.

I remember all these stages like "the terrible twos" or the "threenager" point but I didn't find any of it. Instead, I have loved and embraced every step of being a mom.

Since I'm an older mom, many of my friends are younger than me.

As you can imagine, Jax's classmates' parents are more of the typical age who would have a 6-year old child.

Also, since I have an elementary school child, the parenting issues I encounter are not the same, weightier issues of having a teenager or college-bound child. As the saying goes, "the bigger the child, the bigger the problems."

Finally, because my son is much younger, I am more aware of the kinds of media that influence his generation. I wouldn't know about YouTube channels such as "Ryan's Toy Review," "Azzyland," or "Infinite" without him, nor would I likely do a TikTok dance! But now I do, because Jax does!

So, I absolutely credit Jax for keeping me youthful. I love being an older mom but my age doesn't matter. To him, I'm just Mommy.

12

Take the Risk

"God will not have his work made manifest by cowards." – Ralph Waldo Emerson

I N ORDER NOT TO REMAIN STAGNANT, we have to be willing to step out of our comfort zone and try new things.

Since life is a marathon, not a sprint, I know I must steadily keep moving forward. This is why I continually try to learn new things. According to a recent article I read from Harvard Medical School, learning a new skill can slow cognitive aging.[9]

First, when we learn new skills, our brain chemistry changes. The white matter in our brain (myelin) helps improve performance on a number of tasks. The more we practice a new skill we are learning, the denser the myelin in our brains becomes, which helps us learn even better.[10]

Additionally, learning something new helps us adapt better to

---

[9] Sloan, Matthew. "Back to school: Learning a new skill can slow cognitive aging." *Harvard Health Blog,* 27 April 2016.

[10] Shen, Jason. "The Science of Practice: What Happens When You Learn a New Skill." *Lifehacker.com,* 13 May 2013.

change. It opens up our mind and perceptions, which makes it easier to adapt to the inevitable changes life will undoubtedly bring. Adapting to change is a useful skill in itself, and the more we vary our life experiences and adventures, the easier it is for us to be more flexible and go with the flow.

Another important point I read is that learning new skills could prevent the development of dementia, which has been linked to demyelination of the brain.[11] When we actively learn new skills, we don't give our brains a chance to demyelinate, and our neural pathways are ready for new impulses to travel along them.

As many of you already know, my latest learning experience and biggest change I recently made was moving to the Algarve in Portugal from our home in Southern California. Prior to our move, I had lived in "The OC" for 16 years, after living in New York City. Clearly, there are so many differences between Europe and the USA – European and Portuguese culture, language, foods, currency, and customs, and that's just to start.

I remember the day when Ry had suggested we live abroad. As a Full Stack Software Developer with his own business, Ry has always only needed a computer to do his work. I told him that was the best idea I had heard in a really long time! We were both excited for a new change of scene, and since Ry had never traveled outside of Mexico or ever lived abroad before, it would really be a new learning experience for him. It would be for me, too, but since I had traveled and lived abroad in Europe before, I had an idea of what to expect.

As you can imagine, Ry had more of an adjustment to settling in Portugal than I did. There were a few times when Ry was ready to move back to the States, while I had already settled in and felt at home.

---

[11] Park, Alice. "If You Want to Avoid Dementia, Here's What to Know." *Time,* 24 Feb. 2017.

I thought he was ultimately going to throw in the towel, but, slowly and surely, Ry learned to adapt to his new home, so much so that we extended our resident visa and are staying here longer than planned. In fact, now he loves it here very much, maybe even more than me.

Moreover, I have also made a whole new set of friends here, all from different parts of the world who all speak their own native languages, and of course, I have an entirely different daily routine from the one I had in the USA.

Plus, I am doing different things and learning new skills. For example, I play padel weekly with my dear girlfriends. Padel is a racket sport that combines the elements of tennis, squash and badminton and is very popular in Europe, but I had never even heard of it when I lived in the US.

Another thing I am learning to do is ride a horse. Believe me, I am still scared to do it, but at my last lesson, I was actually galloping.

Taking the risk and doing things that scare me helps eliminate any limits I subconsciously put on my life. Without trying, I will never know so I give myself the opportunity to fail… and learn.

Recently I watched Jax play in a basketball tournament. Many of his teammates are incredible athletes and I see when they do these three-on-three person matches, Jax likes to be a good defender. He is very good at blocking so his opponent won't get the ball. But, when he has to play offense, that's a different story.

During his practices, I remind Jax to go after the ball. Without possession of the ball, you don't have any possibility of taking the shot. Slowly, he is gaining the confidence to try. I was so proud of him during the tournament because he was open to get the ball, dribble it down the court, and take the shot. Although he missed the basket each time, I know that one day soon he will be able to get the point because now he isn't afraid to actually have the ball in his hands.

Before the tournament, Jax would almost seem to be paralyzed when he had the ball, and wouldn't know what to do with it, or he would try to quickly pass the ball to his teammates so he wouldn't be the one in possession of it.

But this time, he finally had the courage to keep it and do something with it. I am such a proud mama!

I think this story illustrates the Ralph Waldo Emerson quote I mentioned at the start of the chapter, and watching my son play basketball reminds me that I, too, have to go after the ball and try. If I don't, I will never get the shot.

As we get older, it is harder to take these risks because we become so comfortable in our routines, or it is too scary to try something new and different and possibly fail at it or be judged. But, it is so important to be continuously evolving.

Some friends and colleagues have commented that it is so brave of us to move to Portugal, but for me, it is all an exciting, big adventure. I love being somewhere new and meeting different people with new energy. Of course, many things are not the same here in Portugal as they are in the US, but I embrace it all. To me, life can become stale and boring when it is the same thing all the time.

A good challenge for all of us is to list our weaknesses and focus on making one of them stronger in one year. You'll want to tell a close friend so you're accountable, but in your quest to diminish a weakness, you'll find that you will have to put yourself outside your comfort zone and learn a new approach.

Anyway, I do believe this kind of thinking – taking risks, embracing new adventures, placing yourself in an entirely different environment, and happily learning new skills – are ways to stay young.

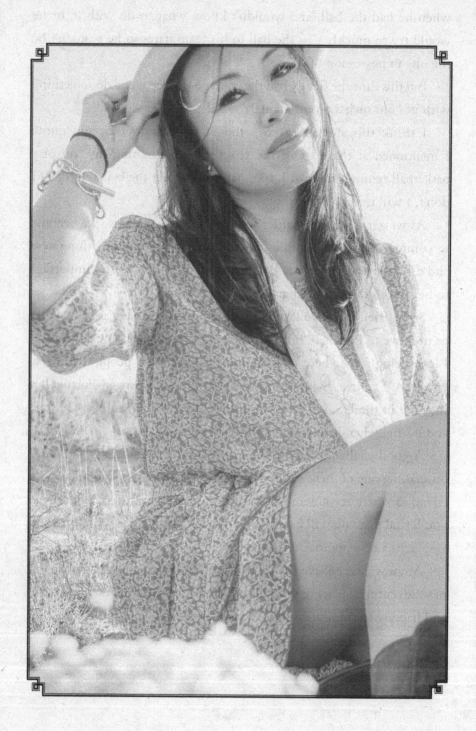

13

Tackle Your Fears

"Too many people are thinking of security instead of opportunity. They seem to be more afraid of life than death."
— James F. Byrnes

S O HOW DO WE OVERCOME FEAR to try new things and take risks? There is no more sure way to fail than to never try.

Fear is not inherently bad or good but a tool we can use to make better decisions. It exists to keep us safe.

Often, however, it is our fear that directs our daily decisions. Fears of scarcity, of the unknown, of others, of harm to loved ones, of abandonment, of not measuring up/being unworthy, of death (just to name a few) can be a root cause of unhappiness, substance abuse, and self-harm.

To tackle it, I try to take fear head on and name the fear. Sometimes merely stating what your fear is gives you the strength to deal with it.

For me, I am afraid that people will judge me. Of course I already know that people will judge me. I am judged on how I look, what I wear, that I am an Ivy League graduate, that I'm not legally married to Ry, that I believe in God. Even though I said earlier that we should stay focused on our goals and not care what others think, for me, it is easier said than done.

I look younger than my age so I rarely say what it is. I know once I do, people will have preconceived notions of what a 49-year old woman should be like, and I do not want to ever feel limited. It makes me sad that as women age, there is implied age discrimination.

According to an article I read in *Forbes*, a landmark 2015 study by three economists concluded that age discrimination in hiring is particularly bad for women.[12]

The study found that the one occupation where the researchers studied both men and women – sales – there was "considerably stronger evidence of discrimination against older women than older men."

There is even an American comedy-drama series, **Younger**, which main plotline is of a 40-year-old divorcee who has to manage her career in a publishing company having faked her identity as a younger woman to get her job. It's an entertaining series but it's just ridiculous that a plotline like that is plausible!

When I feel like fear is having a stronghold on my decisions, I will take the time to be silent and meditate so that I am calm and my breath is even.

I said earlier that meditation is listening to the Universe, and I can usually conjure up and hear more loving and positive thoughts to move forward.

I also like to focus on gratitude. When I am grateful, there is no room for fear in my heart.

For example, what if I was too afraid to admit my actual age and not write this book? Or that I was too scared to open up and share aspects of my life with you? This could have plausibly happened but thankfully,

---

[12] Barnes, Patricia. "Age Discrimination Is A Women's Issue That Women's Groups Tend to Ignore." *Forbes*, 4 July 2019.

I moved past my fear of judgment so I could share this and hopefully, inspire and help many of you.

In doing so, instead of being scared, I am appreciative that I have the opportunity to perhaps provide some wisdom and experience that could really be motivating, useful, and helpful.

There are also times when I feel very strong and confident and then suddenly, I have a fear-based thought creep into my mind. During these times, I have to go back to what I said in Chapter 1 and have the awareness to control my thoughts, eliminate ones that do not serve me, and try to instill a more positive mindset.

Fear is an aging factor, so I try to never make decisions under fear. If needed, I will sleep and meditate on it, and then when I am less emotional, I will have more sound judgment. Actions made under strong emotions are often bad decisions, so I will not rush on a direction if it doesn't feel right.

Learning to handle fear and overcome it is so critical to living a full life, and I intend to live my life to its fullest.

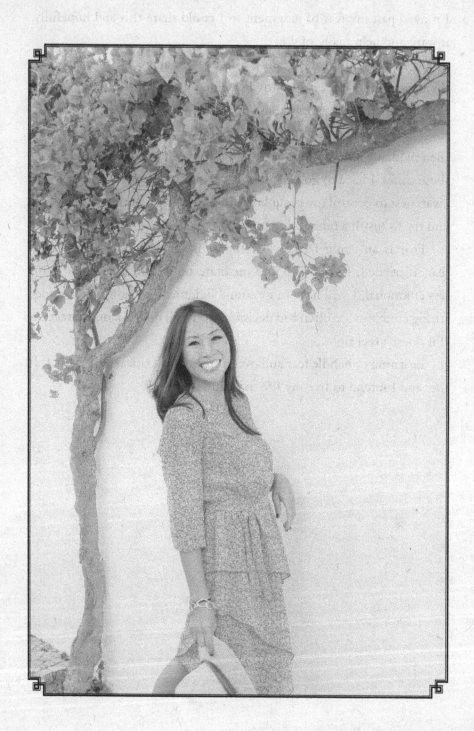

14

Love Who You Are

"Love Yourself." – Jen Sincero, author of *You are a Badass*

IN MY CHILDHOOD HOME, MY PARENTS have a plaque that says: "What you are is God's gift to you. What you make of yourself is your gift to God."

That plaque has consciously and subconsciously directed my entire life.

I also sincerely identify with the "Parable of the Talents." For those that do not know the story, the main lesson and takeaway is that we must make the most of what is given to us and more will be given. But if we squander or do not use what we have, even what we have will be taken away.

At first, it seems like the harshest message. Essentially, the Universe tells us not to waste our lives away, be lazy, and undisciplined, otherwise even our God-given talents will be withdrawn. But, in deeper reading of this lesson, the Universe merely wants us to become the very best versions of ourselves.

To quote the late Kobe Bryant, one of the greatest NBA players of all time, "The most important thing is to try and inspire people so that they can be great in whatever they want to do."

So, how do we do that? This takes some self-introspection. What are you good at? What comes most easily to you? What do you enjoy doing? Then do it and share your gifts with the world.

As Oprah Winfrey has said, "The only courage you will need is the courage to live the life you are meant to."

You may want to ask some close friends or family who you trust on what they think you're good at doing. They can probably provide some insight on what direction is best for you.

For example, for me, I enjoy writing and I like to hang out with my friends. So, being a marketer makes complete sense to me as a career option because I am a natural cheerleader for my friends and I like to inform others all the great things they are doing.

With my marketing clients, I essentially do the same thing. My marketing clients become my friends. Because I care about them, I want them to succeed, so I do my best by telling others what their businesses are all about. Most of this is done through content and writing – via marketing brochures, press releases, case studies, social media posts, and so on.

Everyone has their very own talents, and we must recognize that our talents are just as valuable as any other person's talent.

My sister Pearl is a brilliant mathematician. Economics and advanced equations come very naturally to her, and so she does derivatives on a daily basis in order to help optimize the United States budget and economy.

Doing calculus every day? You would not want me anywhere near that role.

Similarly, my brother RJ is very meticulous and detail-oriented and thus he does very well as a SEO expert, knowing the exact copy and terminology and perfecting the algorithm so that his clients' businesses are easily found online.

We must recognize that we all have our own gifts that could benefit the world!

I believe that once we understand that and love our unique characteristics, and ourselves, it opens us up to doing more for the world. We were all made for a purpose. I think finding and discovering this love within ourselves is the start to doing even greater things.

I realize it is difficult because, for the most part, we all want to fit in and be loved and accepted. But, it is diversity and uniqueness that make the world go around. Sometimes it's easier to hide what we believe is our weirdness and quirkiness, but it is exactly those personality traits that make us endearing. Learning to embrace these characteristics boldly and wholeheartedly make us special.

So many people I know are always trying to project a perfect persona because by doing that, they believe they will receive more acceptance and love by others. But in actuality, it is the opposite case - more people love and cheer for the underdog or the awkward misfit, because there is something more real and relatable about them.

Love of self. I believe that once we can achieve this, it will permeate through your entire being, and it is positively contagious. Your self love will help others find theirs.

15

Enjoy Your Work

"Find a job you enjoy doing, and you will never have
to work a day in your life." – Mark Twain

I WAS TALKING TO MY FRIEND YVETTE Martins (who shot the cover
and the majority of photos in this book) and we agreed that it is
critical to pick a career you love.

Again, it goes back to my feeling that the Universe wants us to
be joyful, and I believe you must be joyful in all things, including the
career you choose for yourself.

When you are vibrating at the highest frequency, not only are
you joyful, but you can be your most creative, and experience greater
personal power and clarity. As Albert Einstein said, "Everything in life
is vibration."

If you dread what you do, then it is time to reconsider what you
are doing.

You cannot be afraid and let fear-based thoughts keep you from
being the best person you can be. Many of us are conditioned to think
that we have to stay in our uninspired jobs because it is steady and stable.
But I am telling you that you have to believe that the money will come

when you do something you love and enjoy and are providing true value to others.

In my case, I am so grateful that I have my own business. Being a marketing consultant suits my life perfectly.

In my younger days, I enjoyed going to a corporate office and working with teams of talented colleagues. It was because of these experiences that I received the foundation for what I now do on my own.

Now that I am a mom, working in a corporate office does not afford me the flexibility I need to live my best life. Since I have always been a very quick and efficient colleague, I know I would feel penalized by being in an office setting with a management team that would expect me to log in certain face-time hours.

Since I often get my best ideas in the early morning or while doing a run, being confined to an office setting doesn't work for me.

I am also incredibly grateful that technology allows me to work remotely with my clients. I save huge amounts of time by not commuting and sitting in traffic. I just open up my computer and then it's off to work I go. Truly, I am even more productive and creative.

Underlying all this is that because I have designed a career that works optimally with my life and I am in control of its trajectory, I do not encounter as much stress as those who feel like they are less in control.

I've already said it numerous times, but stress ages you.

Many of you may know that I had septicemia (or sepsis) in 2009. To this day, I still cannot believe that I was so very sick that I almost died.

The cause of my sepsis was appendicitis. However, my appendix did not burst, it merely tore, and so all the toxins slowly crept into my bloodstream. I remember going to the ER on Saturday with chills on a beautiful 80-degree day, to have the doctor diagnose me with a kidney infection, prescribe Flagyl, and tell me that I should be good by Friday.

So, I went to work every day that next week. I was managing the company's biggest brand at the time and I was recently moved to it and charged to save it after its share had fallen drastically in the last consecutive three years. I felt a lot of pressure to ensure its success, and I was also managing multiple people, including the entire graphic arts department.

I remember when Friday came around, I was still not feeling right; that something was wrong. I returned to the ER on Saturday, had more tests done including an MRI and Ultrasound, and this time, the ER doctor told me, "Promise me you'll go to your OB/GYN first thing Monday morning" since I was complaining of pain in my lower right abdomen.

When Sunday morning arrived, I told Ry, "I don't think I will make it to Monday." I was likely non-responsive, and flowing in and out of a sleep state at that point because Ry pretty much yelled at me and dragged me into the car to take me to Hoag, another hospital in the next town.

My blood pressure was 70/30 and they wheeled me into the hospital right away. I remember an ER nurse yelling "she's septic, she's septic" and telling me, "I don't want to scare you but you have sepsis and we are taking you to ICU." I had no idea what sepsis was so I googled it and the first thing I read was "Most ICU deaths are caused by sepsis."

My appendicitis became peritonitis, which became so bad, it became sepsis. I had to have an emergency appendectomy, and a blood transfusion, and I stayed in the ICU for ten days. Upon release, I still had a PICC line and a home health nurse had to come to my house to administer two sets of IV meds to continue to cleanse my bloodstream for another 10 more days.

It was during my disability leave that I was able to take a step back and examine my life. I had loved the company I worked at for many years (and am still immensely grateful for my time there) but I knew that it was now not a healthy situation for me, and needed to go.

I am intensely loyal so the Universe made the decision for me. When months later, a private equity firm restructured the company and gave me an opportunity to get out, I knew with 100 percent certainty that it was time for me to leave.

So, as scary as it was, I credit my bout with sepsis for opening my eyes up to moving in another direction. As a diligent, A-student, and dutiful daughter of immigrant parents, I just assumed I would be a steady, corporate person my whole life. But after this health scare, I knew I had to find a better way to live.

Anytime you are not feeling calm, centered, and at peace, you open yourself up to aging. According to a 2012 study, published in the journal *PLoS ONE*, researchers measured the length of DNA sections called telomeres, and found that individuals with the most job stress had the shortest telomeres — and when telomeres become too short, the cells can die or become damaged, leading to aging.[13]

I think work-related stress is very prevalent, but it doesn't have to be. The truth is we are all replaceable in the workplace. Of course, no one will be anything like you, but someone can do the fundamentals of the job at hand. Knowing this, it is always important to put your own self and health first. If you are in a place of strength, you can give so much more to others.

---

[13] Ahola K, Sirén I, Kivimäki M, Ripatti S, Aromaa A, Lönnqvist J, et al. (2012) Work-Related Exhaustion and Telomere Length: A Population-Based Study. PLoS ONE 7(7): e40186. https://doi.org/10.1371/journal.pone.0040186

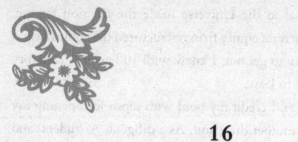

16

Believe

"You don't become what you want, you become what you believe." - Oprah Winfrey

I STARTED THIS BOOK ABOUT OUR THOUGHTS because they are so crucial on how we live our lives.

Honestly, the reason I stay so "preserved" (as a friend of mine once commented about me) is because I believe I am young.

But what we believe about ourselves holds true for all aspects of our life. As Henry Ford famously said, "'Whether you think you can, or you think you can't - you're right."

I can recall a time I was going on a business trip with my friend and colleague Stephanie. She was driving and I was in the passenger seat. All of a sudden, she went over some huge pothole, which caused her tire to deflate right in the middle of the busy I-405 freeway in Los Angeles, with her car stopping instantly.

In most cases, you would think this would cause a multiple-car collision with cars speeding behind us, and inevitably crashing into us. But that didn't happen. I'm fuzzy on the details, but miraculously, all the cars went around us.

When the police arrived, they put up the flares to indicate that we were a stopped car and to go around us, but in those first minutes without police intervention, all the cars just knew to slow down and avoid us.

I will always remember what Stephanie (who is a non-religious person, by the way) said to me: "We're so lucky your guardian angels are always watching over you."

I didn't even think about it, but once she said it, I absolutely agreed that Stephanie's car was spared and we avoided what could have been a very serious accident because angels somehow diverted the traffic.

Many of you may think that is the craziest and most non-sensical story you've ever read, but I believe (really, really believe) that we had divine guidance that day.

I have more interesting stories like that in my life, but I really wanted to illustrate that maybe because I believe in divine guidance, I get it.

As the Bible says, "If you believe, you will receive whatever you ask for in prayer." (Matthew 21:22, NIV).

I think it is my faith that gets me through the most challenging times in my life. I believe that anything negative that happens to me is here to serve a purpose – make me stronger, help me learn a lesson, or give me insight and wisdom, and because I believe this, I have the ability to move forward from tough times.

Of course, I want to be sympathetic to those who face really terrible challenges and don't want to seem glib about these situations. My heart hurts for my close friends who are going through some hard times.

But I want to reinforce the notion that because of my belief system, I am likely to find peace in even the most trying of times.

It is also because of my belief system that I believe that, like Gabby Bernstein, "the Universe has my back."

Many of our beliefs were created when we were young, or possibly passed on through our parents, or even generations before them.

I am not versed enough in psychology to dissect how our preconceived notions become part of us and drive our decision-making, but sometimes we have to question our long-held beliefs if they don't seem to be helping us.

For example, beliefs about money often hold us back.

If you grew up hearing that the only way to make money is to work hard, you may think that you must work hard at (and thus not enjoy) your job because that is the only way to earn riches.

The same goes with aging. Maybe you believe that when you automatically turn 40, you will need bi-focals or readers. I'm not saying that you can will this not to happen, but I do think your body responds to your inner thoughts, and it will more likely happen if you're expecting it.

I think what we believe has such a great impact on all aspects of our life, so let's choose to believe in positive, affirming thoughts.

17

Give, Give, and Give Some More

"Each one must give as he has decided in his heart,
not reluctantly or under compulsion, for God loves a
cheerful giver." (2 Corinthians 9:7, ESV)

I SINCERELY BELIEVE BEING A KIND, GIVING person will keep you young.

In our society, and in the US especially, independent achievement gets the accolades and recognition. We focus on our latest goals, how we can improve ourselves and reach our full potential, our specific pedigrees, our career trajectory, and our own families. Of course, I do this, too.

But, I believe that when we make ourselves the primary focus all the time and are selfish and self-centered, we become too preoccupied with our ego, and I truly think this ages us.

Possessing a "me, me, me, and my own needs/affairs" mentality will only internalize our own issues and problems which will sit inside our bodies and create stress and toxicity.

On the other hand, if you stop thinking about how everything impacts you all the time and start focusing on trying to help and positively affect the lives of others, I believe your light and energy become an external force that radiates.

I agree wholeheartedly with Anne Frank's words: "No one has ever become poor by giving."

I can't even begin to tell you that when I shifted my mindset to that of servant, I felt the world opened up to me and I was in a position to make a greater impact. When I push my ego aside, I actually start thinking bigger.

Moving from "what do I get out of it" to "what can I give" has only opened more doors of opportunity for me. Believe me, if you are always calculating in your head what you can get back in return, it will make you miserable and unsatisfied. Sadly, this kind of thinking is one of lack vs. abundance.

When one gives, they are not worried that they are losing something. They give because they have plenty to give, or believe they have abundant resources. And this feeling of abundance manifests in actual goods!

When I stopped worrying and focusing on my own needs and wants, they decided to fall effortlessly into my lap. Seriously the strangest outcome of sincerely becoming a more giving person is that I started receiving even more!

Case in point: a few years ago, my friend Gail asked me to help her with her conference, The Heart Series. It is now in its 6th year and it is the conference for socially conscious businesses in the US, with noted speakers from companies such as Toms, Feed, Movember, Lululemon, and The Honest Company.

I was very excited to help volunteer and be surrounded by a group of very mindful and conscientious business people whose main mission is to better the world.

I had no goal in mind but to have fun and use my skill sets to help Gail and her co-founder Megan put out the best event possible.

So of course, I did! I made wonderful friends from this experience, met like-minded people like me, and eventually gained the business of one of my favorite clients because of another friend I met at the conference. I really received a tenfold return if not more.

And this is merely one example – I have so, so many more.

But, as the Bible says, you must be a cheerful giver. You must give because you want to give not because you are expecting anything in return. And I can tell you from my own experience, that you will be greatly rewarded.

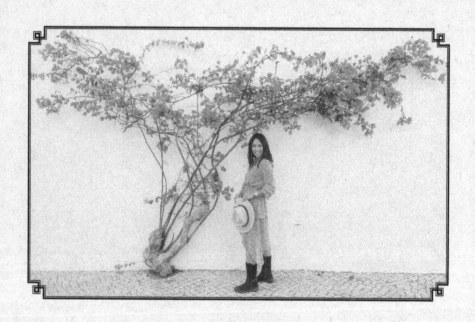

18

Whatever

"Whatever." – Tricia Buenvenida

I AM A DICHOTOMY OF SORTS. YES, I do have a Type-A, overachiever personality (or as Ry tells me, I'm an A++), but there's also the part of me that doesn't really care about the outcome.

My overachiever personality is a by-product of being an immigrant daughter. Since my parents credit their own achievements to breaking out of their poor upbringing in a third world country and creating an "American dream" life for themselves and their children, as a respectful and grateful daughter, I always strive to do more because I want to make my parents proud of me.

Even now that my Dad has passed away, my Dad's legacy of excellence and achievement always influences my life.

But apparently, "whatever" is my favorite word. I laugh because there have been numerous people who have told me this. My dear friend Cindy even gave me a magnet when I was in high school that says "Whatever."

I don't know if that's part of my secret to staying young but maybe it is. I suppose it is conflicting for a typical overachiever who expects certain results. Yet, I'm not really vested in having everything go my way all the time.

Don't get me wrong. I will absolutely give 110% to all my efforts with hopes that the results turn out how I would like, but I am also OK if they don't.

Honestly, if things don't work out like I'd like, then what can I do? I believe that if I gave it my best, then whatever happens after that is out of my control. There are too many other external forces that are in play.

For example, when I applied to Wharton for my MBA, it was my top choice dream school. But, it is extremely competitive to go to this school with only about a 12% acceptance rate, and there are many applicants who apply who have accomplished incredibly amazing things. I could only present my best self with hopes that my best was good enough to be in the matriculating class.

I did not have the best GMAT scores but they were borderline acceptable. I credit strong work experience, good grades, and great recommendation letters for giving me a stronger application. But, I did do two things that helped me stand out from the pool of about 7,000 applicants.

First, since writing is my strong suit, I spent a lot of time perfecting my essays with one of my essays not written in the traditional essay format. I obviously purposely did that so my creative essay could stand out to the admissions committee.

Second, I was able to secure a personal interview on campus. I had met one of the admissions officers at an earlier information session, and when I could not secure a date for a personal interview online, I re-introduced myself at another admissions session, told the officer about my situation, and she graciously gave me her business card and told me to call her to set up an interview. When I took her up on her offer and called the next business day, she gave me an interview time slot on the spot.

Again, I don't know if it was the Universe's forces at work but with that personal interview set, I had all the elements working for me to present myself in the best light possible.

Who knows if I would have been accepted had I not had met and later seen that Admissions officer? Would a missing personal interview in my file be a huge strike in my total application? I think so and I am forever grateful to that officer for giving me that time slot.

Regardless, if I was not accepted to Wharton, I had applied to other fantastic schools and so I knew I would find my place and be fine.

I carry this attitude with all aspects of my life. At the end of the day, I let go and "let God." I believe that if I gave my best effort then whatever happens after that, happens for a purpose, and I can only rest assured that I gave it my all.

I suppose with this understanding that "everything will turn out for the best," I free myself from undue stress and anxiety. So, in a sense, I surrender with great faith knowing that whatever the outcome, it is for the best.

If you don't currently have this ability to surrender, think of all the times in your past when you worried about the outcome. At the end, did it turn out alright? I'm hoping the answer is yes.

Again, you have to believe that you will be OK and if you do end up going in the wrong direction, your instinct will let you know to change course. That's what it does for me. It is because of this faith and assurance that I confidently say "whatever."

CONCLUSION

"Legacy is not leaving something for people. It's leaving something in people." - Peter Strople

So, in a nutshell, these are the "secrets" that have worked for me. I know, they're not earth shattering. Sometimes a little shifting of perspective is all we need.

If you think about it, we'll be lucky if we get to live to 100 years old so our time is very valuable.

For me, I want to a live a life so that when people are around me, they feel loved and accepted to be exactly who they are.

How do you want to make the most of your life and your time here on earth?

From the bottom of my heart, thank you for your time and I sincerely hope some of these tips will work to inspire a more youthful you too.

APPENDIX

Books:

You are a Badass: How to Stop Doubting Your Greatness and Start Living an Awesome Life by Jen Sincero

Think and Grow Rich by Napoleon Hill

The Power is Within You by Louise Hay

Finding Your Own North Star by Martha Beck

Secrets of the Millionaire Mind by T. Harv Eker

As a Man Thinketh by James Allen

Super Attractor: Methods for Manifesting a Life Beyond Your Wildest Dreams by Gabrielle Bernstein

The Master Key System by Charles F. Haanel

Quotes:

"Conquer yourself and the whole universe is yours." - Swami Vivekananda

"Create the highest, grandest vision possible for your life, because you become what you believe." – Oprah Winfrey

"We can change our lives. We can do, have, and be exactly what we wish." – Tony Robbins

"Man's mind stretched to a new idea never goes back to its original dimensions." - Dan Lok

"You need to recognize that your entire life is in your head. It's the way you think. It's the software system for your life computer, and if you want to change your life, it will have to start with the way you think. Choose your thoughts carefully." - T. Harv Eker

"The state of your life is nothing more than a reflection of the state of your mind." — Wayne Dyer

"Every thought we think is creating our future." – Louise Hay